I'm your

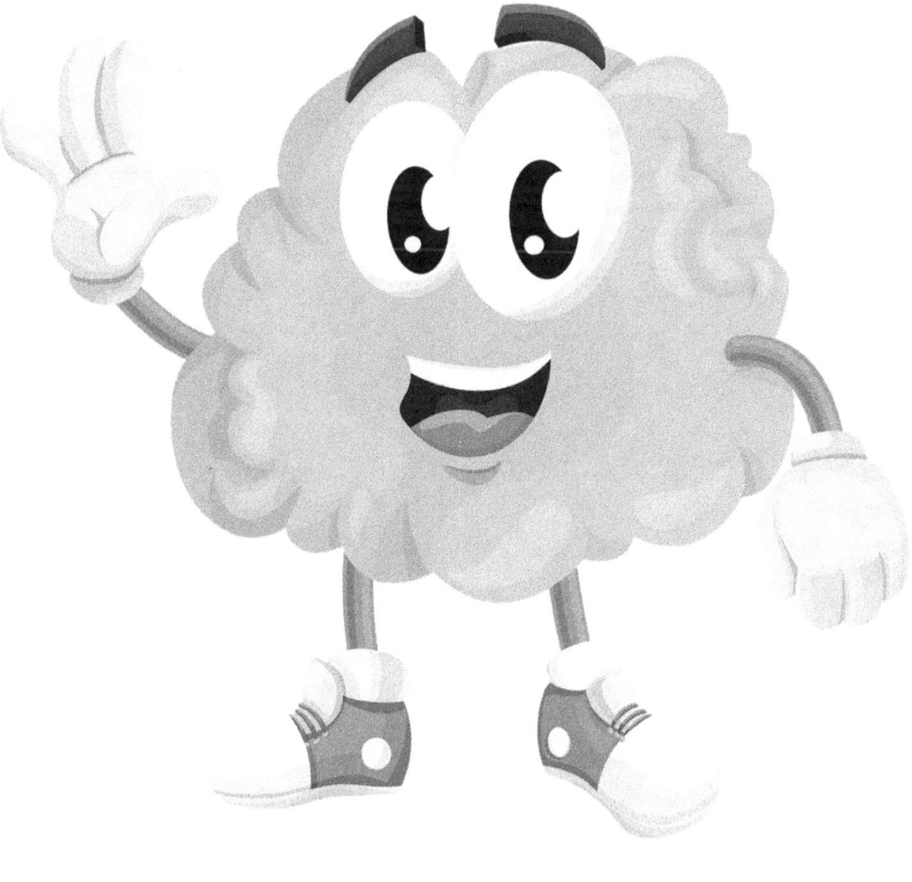

memory

Date:

sun.mon.tue.wed.thu.fri.sat *NOTES*

Date: _____

sun.mon.tue.wed.thu.fri.sat

NOTES

Date:

sun.mon.tue.wed.thu.fri.sat   *NOTES*

Date:

sun.mon.tue.wed.thu.fri.sat

NOTES

Date:

sun.mon.tue.wed.thu.fri.sat *NOTES*

Date:

sun.mon.tue.wed.thu.fri.sat

NOTES

Date:

sun.mon.tue.wed.thu.fri.sat

NOTES

Date:

sun.mon.tue.wed.thu.fri.sat

NOTES

Date:

sun.mon.tue.wed.thu.fri.sat

NOTES

Date: _____

sun.mon.tue.wed.thu.fri.sat

NOTES

Date: _____

sun.mon.tue.wed.thu.fri.sat *NOTES*

Date:

sun.mon.tue.wed.thu.fri.sat

NOTES

Date:

sun.mon.tue.wed.thu.fri.sat   *NOTES*

Date:
sun.mon.tue.wed.thu.fri.sat

NOTES

Date: _____

sun.mon.tue.wed.thu.fri.sat

NOTES

Date:

sun.mon.tue.wed.thu.fri.sat

NOTES

Date: _____

sun.mon.tue.wed.thu.fri.sat

NOTES

Date:

sun.mon.tue.wed.thu.fri.sat

NOTES

Date:

sun.mon.tue.wed.thu.fri.sat

NOTES

Date:

sun.mon.tue.wed.thu.fri.sat

NOTES

Date:

sun.mon.tue.wed.thu.fri.sat *NOTES*

Date:

sun.mon.tue.wed.thu.fri.sat

NOTES

Date: _____

sun.mon.tue.wed.thu.fri.sat   **NOTES**

Date:
sun.mon.tue.wed.thu.fri.sat

NOTES

Date:

sun.mon.tue.wed.thu.fri.sat *NOTES*

Date:

sun.mon.tue.wed.thu.fri.sat

NOTES

Date:

sun.mon.tue.wed.thu.fri.sat   *NOTES*

Date:

sun.mon.tue.wed.thu.fri.sat

NOTES

Date:

sun.mon.tue.wed.thu.fri.sat *NOTES*

Date: _____

sun.mon.tue.wed.thu.fri.sat

NOTES

Date:

sun.mon.tue.wed.thu.fri.sat

NOTES

Date:

sun.mon.tue.wed.thu.fri.sat

NOTES

Date: _____

sun.mon.tue.wed.thu.fri.sat **NOTES**

Date:

sun.mon.tue.wed.thu.fri.sat

NOTES

Date:

sun.mon.tue.wed.thu.fri.sat *NOTES*

Date:

sun.mon.tue.wed.thu.fri.sat

NOTES

Date:

sun.mon.tue.wed.thu.fri.sat

NOTES

Date: _____

sun.mon.tue.wed.thu.fri.sat

NOTES

Date:

sun.mon.tue.wed.thu.fri.sat

NOTES

Date:

sun.mon.tue.wed.thu.fri.sat

NOTES

Date:

sun.mon.tue.wed.thu.fri.sat

NOTES

Date:

sun.mon.tue.wed.thu.fri.sat

NOTES

Date:

sun.mon.tue.wed.thu.fri.sat *NOTES*

Date:

sun.mon.tue.wed.thu.fri.sat

NOTES

Date:

sun.mon.tue.wed.thu.fri.sat *NOTES*

Date:

sun.mon.tue.wed.thu.fri.sat

NOTES

Date:

sun.mon.tue.wed.thu.fri.sat

NOTES

Date:

sun.mon.tue.wed.thu.fri.sat

NOTES

Date:

sun.mon.tue.wed.thu.fri.sat   *NOTES*

Date:

sun.mon.tue.wed.thu.fri.sat

NOTES

Date:

sun.mon.tue.wed.thu.fri.sat

NOTES

Date:

sun.mon.tue.wed.thu.fri.sat

NOTES

Date:

sun.mon.tue.wed.thu.fri.sat

NOTES

Date:

sun.mon.tue.wed.thu.fri.sat

NOTES

Date:

sun.mon.tue.wed.thu.fri.sat   *NOTES*

Date: _____

sun.mon.tue.wed.thu.fri.sat

NOTES

Date:

sun.mon.tue.wed.thu.fri.sat　　　　　　　　　　　　　　　　　　　　　　　*NOTES*

Date:

sun.mon.tue.wed.thu.fri.sat

NOTES

Date: _____

sun.mon.tue.wed.thu.fri.sat   *NOTES*

Date:

sun.mon.tue.wed.thu.fri.sat

NOTES

Date:

sun.mon.tue.wed.thu.fri.sat *NOTES*

Date: _____

sun.mon.tue.wed.thu.fri.sat

NOTES

Date: _____

sun.mon.tue.wed.thu.fri.sat   **NOTES**

Date:

sun.mon.tue.wed.thu.fri.sat

NOTES

Date:

sun.mon.tue.wed.thu.fri.sat

NOTES

Date:

sun.mon.tue.wed.thu.fri.sat

NOTES

Date:

sun.mon.tue.wed.thu.fri.sat

NOTES

Date:

sun.mon.tue.wed.thu.fri.sat

NOTES

Date:

sun.mon.tue.wed.thu.fri.sat   *NOTES*

Date:

sun.mon.tue.wed.thu.fri.sat

NOTES

Date:

sun.mon.tue.wed.thu.fri.sat

NOTES

Date:

sun.mon.tue.wed.thu.fri.sat

NOTES

Date:

sun.mon.tue.wed.thu.fri.sat *NOTES*

Date:

sun.mon.tue.wed.thu.fri.sat

NOTES

Date:

sun.mon.tue.wed.thu.fri.sat

NOTES

Date: _____

sun.mon.tue.wed.thu.fri.sat

NOTES

Date:

sun.mon.tue.wed.thu.fri.sat

NOTES

Date:

sun.mon.tue.wed.thu.fri.sat

NOTES

Date:

sun.mon.tue.wed.thu.fri.sat *NOTES*

Date:

sun.mon.tue.wed.thu.fri.sat

NOTES

Date:

sun.mon.tue.wed.thu.fri.sat   *NOTES*

Date:

sun.mon.tue.wed.thu.fri.sat

NOTES

Date: _____

sun.mon.tue.wed.thu.fri.sat   **NOTES**

Date:

sun.mon.tue.wed.thu.fri.sat

NOTES

Date:

sun.mon.tue.wed.thu.fri.sat

NOTES

Date:

sun.mon.tue.wed.thu.fri.sat

NOTES

Date:

sun.mon.tue.wed.thu.fri.sat

NOTES

Date:

sun.mon.tue.wed.thu.fri.sat

NOTES

Date:

sun.mon.tue.wed.thu.fri.sat

NOTES

Date:

sun.mon.tue.wed.thu.fri.sat

NOTES

Date:

sun.mon.tue.wed.thu.fri.sat   *NOTES*

Date:

sun.mon.tue.wed.thu.fri.sat

NOTES

Date:

sun.mon.tue.wed.thu.fri.sat

NOTES

Date:

sun.mon.tue.wed.thu.fri.sat

NOTES

Date:

sun.mon.tue.wed.thu.fri.sat

NOTES

Date:

sun.mon.tue.wed.thu.fri.sat

NOTES

Date:

sun.mon.tue.wed.thu.fri.sat

NOTES

Date:

sun.mon.tue.wed.thu.fri.sat

NOTES

Date:

sun.mon.tue.wed.thu.fri.sat   *NOTES*

Date:

sun.mon.tue.wed.thu.fri.sat

NOTES

Date:

sun.mon.tue.wed.thu.fri.sat

NOTES

Date:

sun.mon.tue.wed.thu.fri.sat

NOTES

Date:

sun.mon.tue.wed.thu.fri.sat *NOTES*

Date: _____

sun.mon.tue.wed.thu.fri.sat

NOTES

Date:

sun.mon.tue.wed.thu.fri.sat *NOTES*

Date:

sun.mon.tue.wed.thu.fri.sat

NOTES

Date:

sun.mon.tue.wed.thu.fri.sat *NOTES*

www.ingramcontent.com/pod-product-compliance
Lightning Source LLC
Chambersburg PA
CBHW070421220526
45466CB00004B/1502